# Re-challenging and Reintroducing FODMAPS

## A self-help guide to the entire reintroduction phase of the low FODMAP diet

## By Lee Martin RD MSc

W9-BQJ-146

© 2016 by Lee Martin

All rights reserved. No part of this publication may be reproduced, distributed, or transmitted in any form or by any means, including photocopying, recording, or other electronic or mechanical methods, without the prior written permission of the publisher, except in the case of brief quotations embodied in critical reviews and certain other non-commercial uses permitted by copyright law.

**Disclaimer**

This book is based on the most up to date available research and clinical practices on the low FODMAP diet at the time of publication (October, 2015). The book does not replace the advice that should be sought from a qualified health professional. Ideally you should receive a diagnosis of IBS from your doctor and ensure all other causes of your IBS symptoms have been investigated prior to making any changes to your diet. This is particularly important if you are planning to remove gluten from your diet but have not had a screening for coeliac disease. If this statement raises unanswered questions for you then please see your doctor immediately.

# Introduction

The reintroduction phase is the second phase of the three phase low FODMAP diet. Currently you have been following phase one of the low FODMAP diet where you restrict the amount of FODMAPs you consume daily to reduce the severity of your IBS symptoms. This first phase is called the low FODMAP restriction diet and is only meant to be followed for a few weeks (i.e. 2-6 weeks) with the sole aim of reducing symptoms.

The reintroduction phase itself is split into two parts where first you **re-challenge** your tolerance levels to the FODMAPs you avoided during the restriction phase of the low FODMAP diet. This re-challenge part is mainly to help identify which particular single FODMAPs trigger symptoms and what portion size of that FODMAP you can tolerate i.e. small, medium or large portion sizes.

Secondly you **reintroduce** the FODMAPs you can tolerate into your diet and continue to follow a modified low FODMAP diet in the long term to self-manage your IBS symptoms. The reintroducing part is really important for discovering what combination of FODMAPs and what overall load (total amount) of FODMAPs you can eat in a day or week without triggering IBS symptoms. This will be very helpful for planning meals and eating out. It will also help you understand how foods containing more than one type of FODMAP can be included in a long term modified low FODMAP diet without triggering severe symptoms.

The third and final phase of the low FODMAP diet is becoming known as a **modified low FODMAP diet**.  A modified low FODMAP diet provides you with the flexibility to consume FODMAPs but maintain an overall lower level of FODMAPs to aid in the long term self-management of your IBS symptoms (see figure 1).

## Figure 1: The three phases of the low FODMAP diet

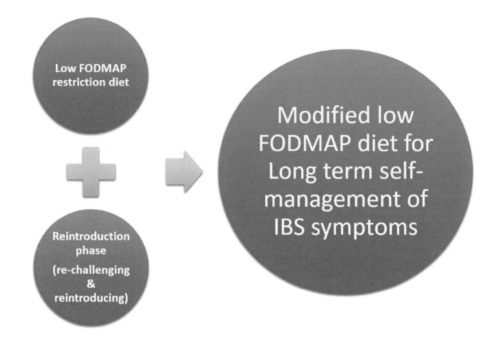

# Aim of the reintroduction phase

The aim of the reintroduction phase is to provide yourself with a better understanding of how FODMAPs affect your IBS symptoms and how you can successfully manage your symptoms in the long term without all the exclusions imposed from a low FODMAP restriction diet.

# How the book will help you

From this point the book will be split into two main sections. The first section will explain how you re-challenge FODMAPs by providing you with a structured protocol and a choice of two methods to follow.  A set of tables which detail the foods containing **individual FODMAPs** to be re-challenged is provided, along with the appropriate portion sizes to consume.

The second section explains the reintroducing part of the reintroduction phase. It outlines how you can attempt to reintroduce FODMAPs back into your diet based on the results you obtain from your re-challenges. This leads to you following a modified low FODMAP diet in the long term. A set of tables of foods that contain **more than one type of FODMAP** is included for reference.

At the end of the book is an extensive Frequently Asked Questions section with many valuable answers to common problems encountered from the reintroduction phase.

# Section 1: Re-challenging FODMAPs

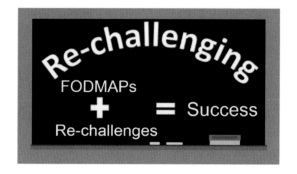

## *Introduction*

This section will explain how you re-challenge FODMAPs by providing you with a structured protocol which allows you to complete the re-challenge process in a systematic way. Please make sure you read the 'rules' and understand the protocol before starting!

## *Before you start*

Please note before you start the re-challenges is it important that you followed the low FODMAP restriction diet correctly and strictly and you have experienced a reduction in your usual IBS symptoms.

Before you start re-challenging ensure you are feeling well and have not just started taking any new medications or are doing anything differently to what you would do normally. For example if you usually smoke then continue to smoke your normal amount, or if you normally drink 3 cups of coffee per day then continue to do this during the re-challenges.

It is best to do the re-challenges in an environment you are comfortable in so you are not stressed as this can affect your symptom response. A comfortable environment can also help keep boost your confidence for trying all the different re-challenges.

## Re-challenging '10 Rules'

1. Always follow the **protocol** (found after the 'rules') and always use the **FODMAP portion sizes of foods tables** (found later in this section) when re-challenging.

2. Always continue to follow a **low FODMAP restriction diet** during the whole re-challenging process.

3. Only once you have re-challenged **all FODMAPs** can you reintroduce them back into your diet. Therefore, for example, even if you find you can tolerate fructose after re-challenging you must still avoid this in your diet until you have completed all the other re-challenges.

4. To follow the protocol you must complete the 3 re-challenges **3 days in a row.**

5. You start with re-challenge 1 which is a small portion size of FODMAP and move onto re-challenge 2 and 3 which **gradually increase the portion size of the FODMAP.**

6. If after any of the 3 re-challenges you only experience **mild symptoms** you should **continue** to the next re-challenge to test the next portion size of FODMAPs.

7. If after any of the 3 re-challenges you experience **severe symptoms** you should **stop** that re-challenge, record your results and enter the 'washout period' (see 'rule' 10)

8. If you feel your symptoms are in-between mild and severe then you will need to make your own decision as to whether you attempt the next FODMAP portion size.

9. You do not need to re-challenge the **large portion size** (re-challenge 3) if it is unrealistic or seems too large for your normal consumption.

10. Each re-challenge is followed by a **'washout period'** of 3 days where you should be free of symptoms before you attempt the next FODMAP re-challenge.

## Re-challenging Protocol

To complete a re-challenge should take 1 week maximum depending on symptoms. This is because there are 3 re-challenge FODMAP portion sizes per food and a 3 day 'washout period' after this. There are 10 re-challenges to complete in total; please see the FODMAP portion size tables for additional instructions.

When deciding on what FODMAP to re-challenge first there are no 'rules'. Usually you will want to re-challenge the foods you missed the most. Often the FODMAP fructans are chosen first as they include wheat bread, garlic and onion which are all popular foods. However it can be easier to start by re-challenging other FODMAPs. As fructans are found in a wide variety of foods you need to re-challenge several foods while for the other FODMAPs you only need one re-challenge. For example the FODMAP GOS (galacto-oligosaccharides) found in chickpeas, or the FODMAP sorbitol found in avocado, can be easier to re-challenge to start with to help you get used to the re-challenge process and discover what FODMAPs are your triggers.

Do not forget to follow the 3 day 'washout period' at the end of each re-challenge whether you experienced any symptoms or not. This is because even if you do not experience any symptoms after re-challenging a large portion size of one FODMAP there may be a carryover effect if the next day you immediately start re-challenging a different FODMAP.

Before starting please remember rule 2 - Always continue to follow a **low FODMAP restriction diet** during the whole re-challenging process!

# Figure 2: Protocol flowchart

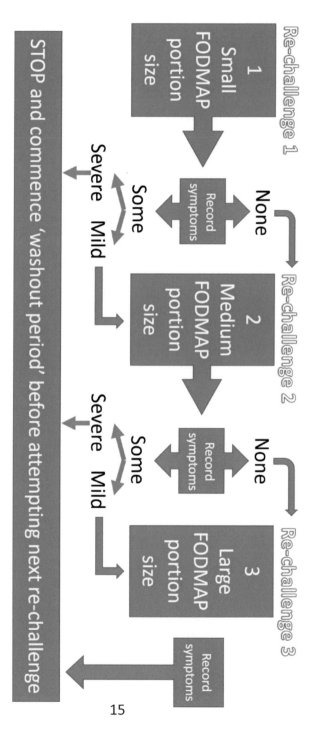

## Re-challenging FODMAP portion sizes

You will notice from the FODMAP portion size tables at the end of this section that the portion sizes are different for different foods. **This is because the portion size relates to the amount of FODMAPs found in the food rather than a typical serving size of that food.** Remember it is not the food you are testing but the amount of FODMAPs found in the food. You do not need to re-challenge the large portion size if it is unrealistic or seems too large for your normal consumption. The amount of FODMAPs found in the food in relation to the portion size is as follows:

**Small portion size = moderate amount of FODMAPs**

**Medium portion size = high amount of FODMAPs**

**Large portion size = very high amount of FODMAPs**

## Understanding your results

It is a good idea to keep a **symptom diary** when re-challenging FODMAPs. This way you can easily record your symptoms and can look back at the diary for reference. You do not need to keep a **food**

**and symptom** diary as you are only re-challenging one FODMAP at a time but you can if you wish. The diary can simply be written down or there are also some useful apps available, either free or fairly cheap, which can help record your symptoms and your stool movements. For example just search for 'IBS' or 'IBS diary' in your app store to find one you like. Remember symptoms may appear several hours later for some or quicker for others. This will depend on your individual gut transit time and other factors.

If you are unsure as to whether or not a symptom was triggered due to the FODMAP you were re-challenging or let's say because you were having a stressful or hectic day, then you can test the same FODMAP portion size again (or occasionally a slightly smaller amount) to double check.

The whole point in recording your symptoms and relating it to the amount of FODMAPs consumed is to work out what portion size of FODMAPS you can tolerate. For example why would you avoid sorbitol completely when you can tolerate a small amount and that way can still eat small amounts of healthy and tasty vegetables such as broccoli and avocado?

## FODMAP tolerance

To help determine what the results from your re-challenges mean for you practically when reintroducing FODMAPs back into your diet please refer to Figure 3; the 'FODMAP Tolerance table'. This table describes the types of tolerance you have to different FODMAPs at the portion sizes consumed during the re-challenges.  It is worth noting that your tolerance to FODMAPs can change over time. Therefore you may wish to re-challenge a particular FODMAP again in the future. This is especially beneficial for those of you who may find that several FODMAPs affect your symptoms as in the future you may be able to consume the foods you currently need to restrict.

# Figure 3: FODMAP Tolerance Table

| FODMAP portion size that symptoms occurred | Practical outcome |
|---|---|
| ☐ Small portion size | ☐ This FODMAP is a major trigger of your IBS symptoms and should be restricted |
| ☐ Medium portion size | ☐ You can eat this FODMAP in moderation |
| ☐ Large portion size | ☐ Generally you can eat this FODMAP but avoid large portion sizes |

# Alternative protocol

Although this book describes the most accepted protocol for re-challenging FODMAPs over a 3 consecutive day period there is an alternative method. The alternative protocol involves re-challenging FODMAPs over a 5 day period with a one day 'rest period' in-between the re-challenges. This alternative protocol is shown in Figure 4.

You still need to follow all the re-challenging 'rules' and the instructions from the original protocol but the only difference is after each portion size re-challenge you do not then re-challenge a larger portion size the next day. Instead you just continue with your low FODMAP diet for a day and then the day after that start to re-challenge the next FODMAP portion size.

This may be beneficial for those who are anxious about re-challenging FODMAPs 3 days in a row as in the original protocol. The potential downside is that it does make the process longer as you are including an extra 2 'rest periods' making each re-challenge

8 days long including the washout period rather than 6. Only choose

this alternative protocol if the speed of the original protocol

concerns you.

# Figure 4: Alternative protocol

| Day 1 | Day 2 | Day 3 | Day 4 | Day 5 | Day 6, 7 & 8* |
|---|---|---|---|---|---|
| Re-challenge 1 | 'rest day' | Re-challenge 2 | 'rest day' | Re-challenge 3 | Commence 'washout period' |
| Small portion size | LFD | Medium portion size | LFD | Large portion size | LFD |

LFD in this table represents the Low FODMAP restriction diet

(remember to follow a LFD throughout all re-challenges)


* washout period may be longer than 3 days depending on

symptom response after re-challenge 3

# Tables: Re-challenge FODMAP Portion Sizes of Foods

The following tables provide an overview of the foods that only contain one **individual FODMAP** and gives you serving suggestions based on the type of portion size you should re-challenge with.

## *GOS (Galacto-oligosaccharides)*

All of the foods in this table only contain high amounts of the FODMAP GOS. **You only need to choose one food to re-challenge.** Always choose an average or medium sized fruit or vegetable unless stated otherwise. Stick to the same food for the duration of the 3 day re-challenge.

## GOS Re-Challenge Table

| Re-challenge Food | Small portion size | Medium portion size | Large portion size |
|---|---|---|---|
| Almonds | 15 nuts | 20 nuts | 25 nuts |
| Black beans (canned) | 2 tablespoons | 4 tablespoons | 6 tablespoons |
| Cassava | 100g / 3oz | 150g / 5oz | 200g / 7oz |
| Chick peas (canned) | 2 tablespoons | 4 tablespoons | 6 tablespoons |
| Custard apple | ¼ of an apple | ½ an apple | 1 whole apple |
| Karela | ¼ of a karela | ½ a karela | 1 whole karela |
| Peas | 2 tablespoons | 4 tablespoons | 6 tablespoons |

For the GOS re-challenge there are only a few foods that contain GOS as the only FODMAP. If you do not like these foods but usually consume one or some of the additional foods listed below then use one of these as your re-challenge instead and stick to the portion sizes detailed above for the pulses and legumes i.e. 2,4 and 6 tablespoons.

The reason why these foods are not in the table above is because they also contain small amounts of fructans as well as GOS (see the reintroducing and combining FODMAPs tables at the end of section 2).

Additional foods: Borlotti beans (canned), Butter beans (canned), Haricot beans (boiled), Lentils (canned), Lentils (green or red, boiled), Lima beans (boiled), Mung beans (boiled), Red kidney beans, Soya beans (boiled), Split peas (boiled).

## *Fructans*

**You will need to re-challenge several fructan containing foods as this FODMAP is found in many different fruits and vegetables at varying amounts and also in wheat.  Therefore the fructans section includes 3 tables and you re-challenge one or two different foods per table.**

## Fructan Vegetables

All of the foods in this table only contain high amounts of the FODMAP fructans. **You need to re-challenge two different vegetables containing fructans.**  Always choose an average or medium sized fruit or vegetable unless stated otherwise. Stick to the same food for the duration of the 3 day re-challenge.

## Fructan Vegetables Re-Challenge Table

| Re-challenge Food | Small portion size | Medium portion size | Large portion size |
|---|---|---|---|
| Garlic _(circled)_ | ¼ of a clove *OR* | ½ a clove | 1 whole clove |
| Leek (white bulb) | ¼ of a leek | ½ a leek | 1 whole leek |
| Okra | 8 pods | 12 pods | 16 pods |
| Onion (red or white) _(circled)_ | ¼ of an onion *OR* | ½ an onion *OR* | 1 whole onion *never eat* |
| Savoy cabbage | 50g / 2oz | 80g/3oz | 140g / 5oz |
| Shallot onions | ½ a shallot | 1 whole shallot | 2 whole shallots |
| Spring onion (white bulb) | ½ a spring onion bulb | 1 whole spring onion bulb | 2 spring onion bulbs |

## Fructan Fruits

All of the foods in this table only contain high amounts of the FODMAP fructans. **You only need to choose one fruit containing fructans to re-challenge.** Always choose an average or medium sized fruit or vegetable unless stated otherwise. Stick to the same food for the duration of the 3 day re-challenge.

Fructan Fruits Re-Challenge Table

| Re-challenge Food | Small portion size | Medium portion size | Large portion size |
|---|---|---|---|
| Grapefruit | 100g / 3oz | 200g / 7oz | 300g / 10oz |
| Persimmon | ¼ of a persimmon | ½ a persimmon | 1 whole persimmon |
| Pomegranate seeds | ½ a small pomegranate | 1 small pomegranate | 2 small pomegranate |
| Rambutan | 4 rambutans | 6 rambutans | 8 rambutans |
| Dried cranberries | 2 tablespoons | 4 tablespoons | 6 tablespoons |
| Dried currants | 1 tablespoon | 2 tablespoons | 4 tablespoons |
| Dried dates | 1 dried date | 2 dried dates | 4 dried dates |
| Dried figs | 1 dried fig | 2 dried figs | 4 dried figs |
| Dried Goji berries | 1 tablespoon | 2 tablespoons | 4 tablespoons |
| Dried mango | 1 piece (5g) | 2 pieces | 4 pieces |
| Dried papaya | 2 pieces (10g) | 3 pieces | 4 pieces |
| Dried pineapple | 1 piece (25g) | 2 pieces | 4 pieces |
| Raisins | 1 tablespoon | 2 tablespoons | 4 tablespoons |

# Fructan Bread, cereals and grains

All of the foods in this table only contain high amounts of the FODMAP fructans. **You need to re-challenge two different foods containing fructans.** Stick to the same food for the duration of the 3 day re-challenge.

Fructan Bread, Cereal and Grains Re-Challenge Table

| Re-challenge Food | Small portion size | Medium portion size | Large portion size |
|---|---|---|---|
| Breakfast Cereals | | | |
| Barley flakes | 20g / ½oz | 40g / 1oz | 60g / 2oz |
| Corn flakes | 30g / 1oz | 45g / 1 ½oz | 60g / 2oz |
| Oats* | 50g / 2oz | 100g / 3oz | 150g / 5oz |
| Rice Krispies | 30g / 1oz | 45g / 1 ½oz | 60g / 2oz |
| Spelt flakes | 20g / ½oz | 40g / 1oz | 60g / 2oz |
| Wheat bran | 1 tablespoon (10g) | 2 tablespoons | 3 tablespoons |
| Bread | | | |
| Pumpernickel | 1 slice (50g) | 2 slices | 3 slices |
| White wheat* | 1 slice (25g) | 2 slices | 3 slices |
| Wholegrain wheat* | 1 slice (25g) | 2 slices | 3 slices |
| Cooked grains | | | |
| Buckwheat kernels | 50g / 2oz | 100g / 3oz | 150g / 5oz |
| Cous cous (wheat) | 50g / 2oz | 100g / 3oz | 150g / 5oz |
| Spelt pasta | 100g / 3oz | 150g / 5oz | 200g / 7oz |
| Wheat pasta | 100g / 3oz | 150g / 5oz | 200g / 7oz |

\* These foods also contain the FODMAP GOS but are suitable for re-challenging fructans

## *Fructose*

All of the foods in this table only contain high amounts of the FODMAP fructose. **You only need to choose one food to re-challenge.** Always choose an average or medium sized fruit or vegetable unless stated otherwise. Stick to the same food for the duration of the 3 day re-challenge.

Fructose Re-Challenge Table

| *Re-challenge Food* | *Small portion size* | *Medium portion size* | *Large portion size* |
|---|---|---|---|
| Boysenberry | 5 berries | 10 berries | 15 berries |
| Broad Beans | 25g / 1oz | 50g / 2oz | 100g / 3oz |
| Canned tomatoes | ½ can (200g) | 1 can | 1 ½ cans |
| Feijoa | ½ a small | 1 small | 2 small |
| Fresh Figs | ½ a medium | 1 medium | 2 medium |
| Honey | 1 teaspoon | 1 tablespoon | 2 tablespoons |
| Mango NO GAS Bloating pain strange bowls movements | ¼ of a medium sized | ½ a medium sized | 1 medium sized |
| Sugar snap peas | 15g / ½oz | 30g / 1oz | 60g / 2oz |
| Sundried tomatoes | 4 pieces | 8 pieces | 12 pieces |
| Tamarillo | ½ a medium | 1 medium | 2 medium |

# Lactose

All of the foods in this table only contain high amounts of the FODMAP lactose. **You only need to choose one food to re-challenge.** Stick to the same food for the duration of the 3 day re-challenge.

Lactose Re-Challenge Table

| Re-challenge Food | Small portion size | Medium portion size | Large portion size |
| --- | --- | --- | --- |
| Cream / Sour cream | 60ml | 120ml | 180ml |
| Cream cheese | 40g / 1oz | 80g / 2oz | 120g / 4oz |
| Halloumi | 50g / 2oz | 100g / 3oz | 200g / 7oz |
| Ice cream* | 1 scoop | 2 scoops | 3 scoops |
| Milk (including evaporated or buttermilk) | 125ml | 250ml | 375ml |
| Milk / white chocolate (see note) | 30g / 1oz | 60g / 2oz | 90g / 3oz |
| Ricotta cheese | 80g / 3oz | 160g / 5oz | 240g / 8oz |
| Yoghurt* | 60g / 2oz | 125g / 4oz | 250g / 8oz |

*Handwritten annotations: "Milk / white" is circled; "Caused diarrhea" is written across the Milk / white chocolate row.*

*check label for added high FODMAP ingredients e.g. fructose, inulin, sorbitol etc.

Note: chocolate is not a sensible test. However if you feel chocolate may trigger symptoms and it is something you do consume regularly then these portion sizes can help you test your tolerance levels to the lactose in the milk added to these products.

## Polyols: Mannitol

All of the foods in this table only contain high amounts of the FODMAP mannitol. **You only need to choose one food to re-challenge.** Always choose an average or medium sized fruit or vegetable unless stated otherwise. Stick to the same food for the duration of the 3 day re-challenge.

Mannitol Re-Challenge Table

| Re-challenge Food | Small portion size | Medium portion size | Large portion size |
|---|---|---|---|
| Cauliflower | 30g / 1oz | 60g / 2oz | 90g / 3oz |
| Celery | ¼ of a stick | ½ a stick | 1 stick |
| Sweet potato | 100g / 3oz | 150g / 5oz | 200g / 7oz |

## *Polyols: Sorbitol*

All of the foods in this table only contain high amounts of the FODMAP sorbitol. **You only need to choose one food to re-challenge.** Always choose an average or medium sized fruit or vegetable unless stated otherwise. Stick to the same food for the duration of the 3 day re-challenge.

Sorbitol Re-Challenge Table

| Re-challenge Food | Small portion size | Medium portion size | Large portion size |
|---|---|---|---|
| Avocado | ¼ of an avocado | ½ an avocado | 1 whole avocado |
| Blackberry | 3 berries | 5 berries | 10 berries |
| Broccoli | 60g / 2oz | 120g / 4oz | 180g / 6oz |
| Fresh Coconut | 100g / 3oz | 150g / 5oz | 200g / 7oz |
| Lychee | 5 lychees | 10 lychees | 15 lychees |
| Peach (yellow only) | ¼ of yellow peach | ½ of yellow peach | 1 whole peach |

# Section 2: Reintroducing FODMAPS

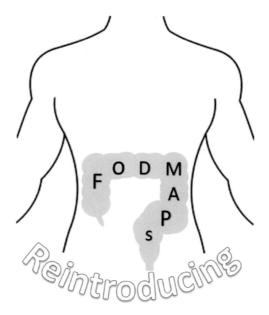

After completing the re-challenges you should have a better

understanding of which FODMAPs are the main triggers of your

symptoms and in what portion sizes you can consume them without

getting symptoms. This helps to define your **FODMAP tolerance**

**level** to individual FODMAPs and everyone will have a different

tolerance level. The next stage is to reintroduce the FODMAPs back

into your diet at a tolerance level that doesn't trigger symptoms.

Once you start reintroducing and combining FODMAPS you need to consider your own individual **FODMAP threshold** for more than one FODMAP. Your FODMAP threshold will help you understand how many FODMAPs you can combine before you go over the threshold and are no longer able to tolerate FODMAPs and experience symptoms.

The vast majority of people who complete the re-challenges and reintroduce FODMAPs follow a **modified low FODMAP diet** in the long term. A modified low FODMAP diet means you can eat and enjoy high FODMAP foods in moderation without going over your FODMAP threshold. This allows you to self-manage your symptoms in the long term without the need to follow a very restricted diet.

### *Discovering your FODMAP threshold*

Your FODMAP tolerance level will be tested as you start to combine different FODMAPs. If you look at Figure 5 it provides an example of reintroducing and combining FODMAPs. The figure explains how you can go over your FODMAP threshold and therefore no longer tolerate FODMAPs.

Discovering your own FODMAP threshold and tolerance levels to a combination of FODMAPs is basically a trial and error process. If you gradually increase your consumption of FODMAPs and monitor your symptoms it will help you understand your tolerance levels easier. Take a look at the tips section and case studies to help you get going.

There are many high FODMAP foods that contain more than one FODMAP and a list of these is provided at the end of this section to help guide you in choosing your FODMAP combinations. These tables are provided to show the FODMAP content of foods so when you are planning your meals you are aware how many different FODMAPs you are combining.

*Figure 5: Example of reintroducing and combining FODMAPs*

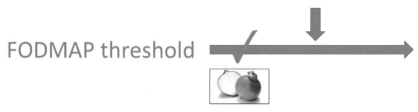

FODMAP threshold

## 1 high FODMAP Food Well under threshold

Example: Your FODMAP threshold is not reached when you eat one high FODMAP food.

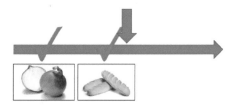

FODMAP threshold

## 2 high FODMAP Foods Just under threshold

Example: You have almost reached your FODMAP threshold when consuming more than one food source of fructans.

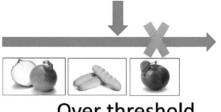

FODMAP threshold

## 3 high FODMAP Foods          Over threshold

Example: Combining the apple which contains more than one FODMAP with other high FODMAP foods has pushed you over your threshold and you can no longer tolerate these FODMAPs.

This final example can apply to foods eaten at the same meal e.g. a baguette for lunch with onion salad and an apple. Or during the course of the same day e.g. baguette for lunch, apple on the way home from work and onion in your dinner meal. It can also apply to larger portions of these foods eaten over more than one day e.g. you have an onion in a stir fry on Monday, a baguette for lunch on Tuesday and an apple crumble for pudding on Wednesday.

**Everybody will have different FODMAP thresholds. The only way to find out yours is to reintroduce FODMAPs.**

## *Reintroducing Tips*

- Reintroducing FODMAPs is not an exact science, so please remember this when trialling!

- You need to use your results from the re-challenges and some common sense to successfully reintroduce FODMAPs without triggering severe symptoms.

- When choosing foods to combine think about your normal meal pattern and what sort of foods and meals you want to eat regularly.

- Gradually increase your overall consumption of FODMAPs and monitor your symptoms. This will help you understand where your FODMAP threshold is and ensure you can tolerate the FODMAPs you are eating.

- Remember the more FODMAPs you consume the more likely you are to go over your threshold. For example a pasta meal including mushrooms, onions and garlic is much more likely to trigger symptoms than a pasta meal including green beans, fennel and garlic.

- Your FODMAP threshold can be reached over the course of one meal, one day or even over several days. It all depends on the amount of FODMAPs consumed and your own tolerance levels. Once the reintroducing of FODMAPs is completed you will know if you can eat FODMAPs every day, or consume FODMAPs every other day, or if you can only consume FODMAPs a couple of times a week before you trigger symptoms.

Here are a couple of 'case studies' to provide a practical example.

## Case study: John

After his re-challenges John found he can tolerate all FODMAPs in isolation at large portion sizes. However when he combined them in the same meal he went over his FODMAP threshold and symptoms occurred.

John is someone who has a 'medium' FODMAP threshold. This means that for John to control his symptoms he should only have a small amount of FODMAPs in his meals i.e. he only consumes one FODMAP per meal with the rest of the meal being low FODMAP. He also needs to be aware that if he consumes several different FODMAPs within the same day he might experience symptoms. Therefore John will follow a modified low FODMAP diet in the long term.


## Case study: Tracy

Tracy only found that lactose was a problem after her re-challenges so she only consumes small amounts of lactose every day and uses alternative milks rather than dairy milk. When she combined

FODMAPs she initially didn't find any problems but after a few weeks started to get symptoms again.

Tracy is someone who has a 'high' FODMAP threshold but an intolerance to lactose. This means that for Tracy she needs to be aware of her FODMAP intake over several days rather than on individual days. She already limits her lactose intake but she needs to remember not to have too many FODMAPs several days in a row as this will trigger her symptoms. Practically it would be good for Tracy to have one or two low FODMAP days per week to prevent her going over her FODMAP threshold. Therefore Tracy will follow a modified low FODMAP diet in the long term.

## Case study: Brian

Brian experienced symptoms with most FODMAPs at medium portion sizes when re-challenging. As he reintroduced and combined FODMAPs he found his symptoms started to get worse. Brian is someone who has a 'low' FODMAP threshold. This means that for Brian he can only consume small amounts of FODMAPs per week without triggering symptoms. Practically this means Brian will only be able to have one or two FODMAPs during the whole day and if he is stressed or other things are affecting his symptoms he may only be able to have a few FODMAP containing foods during the whole week. Therefore Brian will follow a modified low FODMAP diet in the long term.

## Case study: Jane

Jane completed all the re-challenges without any symptoms. She started reintroducing FODMAPs and again did not experience any symptoms. However since doing the low FODMAP diet Jane has found that she tends to eat less onion, garlic and wheat than in her previous normal diet. Jane now says she is eating a normal diet after completing the reintroduction phase of the low FODMAP diet. With Jane her previous diet was only slightly too high in FODMAPs for her FODMAP threshold. Now she has reduced her overall intake of FODMAPs her symptoms have stopped. Although Jane feels she is now eating a normal diet she has reduced her intake of fructans from onion, garlic and wheat and could be considered to be

following an adapted low FODMAP diet too.

# Tables: Reintroducing and combining FODMAPs

## *Fruits*

All of the foods in this table contain high amounts of **more than one FODMAP**.  The portion size relates to an average or medium sized fruit unless stated otherwise. As you can see most fruits contain sorbitol plus one or two other FODMAPs.

**You do not need to re-challenge these foods, the table is for reference and guidance only.**

| Food | Portion size | FODMAPs | | | |
|---|---|---|---|---|---|
| | | Fruc-tose | Sorb | Mann | Fruc-tans |
| Apples | 1 whole apple | X | X | | |
| Apricots | 2 whole apricots | | X | | X |
| Cherries | >6 whole cherries | X | X | | |
| Nectarines | ½ a nectarine | | X | | X |
| Peach (clingstone) | ½ a peach | | X | X | |
| Peach (white) | ½ a peach | | X | | X |
| Pears | ½ a pear | X | X | | |
| Plums | 1 whole plum | | X | | X |
| Prunes | 4 whole prunes | | X | | X |
| Sultanas | 1 tablespoon | X | | | X |
| Watermelon | 1 thick slice (300g) | X | | X | X |
| Dried apple | 2 tablespoons | X | X | | |
| Dried apricot | 2 tablespoons | | X | | X |
| Dried pear | 2 tablespoons | X | X | | |

# Vegetables

All of the foods in this table contain high amounts of more than one FODMAP.  The portion size relates to an average or medium sized vegetable unless stated otherwise.

**You do not need to re-challenge these foods, the table is for reference and to help you reintroduce and combine foods.**

| Food | Portion | FODMAPs | | | | |
| --- | --- | --- | --- | --- | --- | --- |
| | | Fruc-tose | Sorb | Mann | Fruc-tans | GOS |
| Asparagus | >4 spears | X | | | X | X |
| Beetroot | 4 slices (50g) | | | | X | X |
| Butternut squash | 100g | | | X | | X |
| Corn on the cob | 1 whole cob | | X | | | X |
| Mange Tout | 10 pods | | | X | X | X |
| Mushrooms | 80g | | | X | X | |
| Snow peas | 10 pods | | | X | X | X |

## Beans, lentils, nuts and seeds

All of the foods in this table contain high amounts of more than one FODMAP. As you can see all pulses, legumes and nuts listed contain the oligosaccharides GOS and fructans and no other FODMAPs.

**You do not need to re-challenge these foods, the table is for reference and to help you reintroduce and combine foods.**

| Food | Portion size | FODMAPs | |
| --- | --- | --- | --- |
| | | Fructans | GOS |
| Cashew nuts | 20 nuts | X | X |
| Egusi seeds | 4 tablespoons | X | X |
| Hazelnuts | 20 nuts | X | X |
| Pistachio nuts | 15 nuts | X | X |
| Black beans (boiled) | 3 tablespoons | X | X |
| Borlotti beans (canned) | 3 tablespoons | X | X |
| Butter beans (canned) | 4 tablespoons | X | X |
| Haricot beans (boiled) | 3 tablespoons | X | X |
| Lentils (green/red boiled) | 4 tablespoons | X | X |
| Lima beans (boiled) | 4 tablespoons | X | X |
| Mung beans (boiled) | 6 tablespoons | X | X |
| Red kidney beans (boiled) | 3 tablespoons | X | X |
| Soya beans (boiled) | 3 tablespoons | X | X |
| Split peas (boiled) | 3 tablespoons | X | X |

# Bread, cereals and grains

All of the foods in this table contain high amounts of more than one

FODMAP.

**You do not need to re-challenge these foods, the table is for**

**reference and to help you reintroduce and combine foods.**

|  |  | FODMAPs | | |
| --- | --- | --- | --- | --- |
| Food | Portion size | Fructose | Fructans | GOS |
| Bread |  |  |  |  |
| Dark rye bread | 2 slices | X | X | X |
| Rye bread | 2 slices | X | X | X |

Cereals

| Wheat bran pellets | 30g | X | X |  |
| --- | --- | --- | --- | --- |
| Wheat grain biscuits | 2 biscuits |  | X | X |

Cooked Grains

| Freekeh | 100g |  | X | X |
| --- | --- | --- | --- | --- |
| Wheat noodles | 100g | X | X |  |

# Final thoughts

## Perceptions and food obsessions

It is important not to overlook the gut brain interaction when it comes to reintroducing. If you have trepidation regarding the reintroduction phase then before each re-challenge please ask yourself this question:

**Is it the FODMAP or is it the thought of eating the FODMAP that causes my increased symptoms?**

If anxiety about re-challenging a FODMAP is high then read your results with caution. Follow the instructions laid out in this book. By gradually increasing your portion sizes in a systematic way the process can help you gain more control and understand your IBS.

IBS is a complex condition with many attributing factors. The low FODMAP diet has been successful for many people in identifying the main food triggers of symptoms, but it is important to be realistic that it may not remove all your symptoms. We can all still experience stomach discomfort in stressful situations or even when we have consumed too much food.

There is a risk of becoming obsessed by the foods high in FODMAPs and their apparent association with every symptom you experience. This is an unhealthy negative view and it is important that perspective is maintained regarding your IBS symptoms, your environment, the food you are eating, and your own wellbeing.

**Best of luck and remember the low FODMAP diet is not a 'cure' for your IBS but a means to feeling in control. Therefore giving you a healthy mind and a content heart.**

# FODMAP Reintroduction Phase FAQ

*Regarding the FODMAP portion sizes for the third re-challenge, what if I would never eat the portion size of food you are supposed to test, for example broccoli?*

This is where a bit of common sense is needed. What is the point of eating a larger portion size of a food than you ever really would? The answer, of course, is there isn't. The re-challenges should be as realistic as possible i.e. they should represent how you would normally eat the food. Using the question above as an example; if you chose to use broccoli as a re-challenge for the FODMAP sorbitol, on the first re-challenge you would eat approximately 60g, second re-challenge approx. 120g and on the third approx. 180g. Healthy eating guidelines recommend that one normal portion of fruit or vegetables is classed as 80g. Therefore by eating 180g you can consider this a large portion size. If you love broccoli then fine eat 180g and assess your symptoms but if you would never eat this amount of broccoli on a regular basis then don't.  The same rule can be applied to any of the food re-challenges.  Bread contains the FODMAP fructans and is a re-challenged using 1 slice, 2 slices and 3 slices over the three re-challenges.  Although if you don't normally eat 3 slices of bread in one go then why test 3 slices of bread?  Just stop after the second re-challenge and keep it realistic. However if you do normally eat 3 slices of bread spread throughout the day (e.g. 1 slice at breakfast and two at lunch) then you should re-challenge bread in this way rather than eating it all in one go. Having the same food a couple of times a day makes things slightly more complicated but it would still be a perfectly acceptable re-challenge if this is what you would normally do.  The benefit of doing the third re-challenge is it will help you understand your tolerance level to the larger portion size of the individual FODMAP you are testing.

*If I do not like mango or honey for the fructose challenge (for example) can you use any of the other fructose foods e.g. sugar snap peas? And if so how much would you start with to re-challenge?*

For the re-challenges you can use any food that contains a high amount of **one specific FODMAP.** In the case of fructose this includes (mango & honey) boysenberry, fresh figs, sugar snap peas and others. Please note many fruits contain fructose and if eaten in large quantities will contain enough excess fructose to be classed as high FODMAP. Other examples of a suitable fructose re-challenge is canned tomatoes (over 180g or roughly half a can) or sundried tomatoes (over 20g or 5 pieces). Perhaps sundried tomatoes are easy to try. Therefore for your first re-challenge you would start with 4 sundried tomatoes and assess your symptoms and then for the next re-challenge have 8 sundried tomatoes and for the third re-challenge have 12 sundried tomatoes. Remember if you would not normally eat 12 sundried tomatoes then do not attempt the third challenge.

***If I am still having symptoms should I start the***

***reintroduction phase? When do I know my symptoms***

***are low enough to start the next re-challenge?***

Ideally you would need at least 3 days being 'symptom free' before

you start the reintroduction phase. This rule is also applicable to

between different re-challenges i.e. you should not have symptoms

for 3 days before starting a re-challenge. This is why there is the

'washout period' of 3 days after each re-challenge.  It is best to stick

to this rule as best as you can otherwise trying to work out what

FODMAP is the cause of the symptoms will become more confusing.

However being 'symptom free' for 3 days may be difficult for some.

If you were still experiencing symptoms during the low FODMAP

restriction diet but these were at a lower level than when you

started then this lower level of symptoms may have to be what you

class as being 'symptom free'. When you then re-challenge a

FODMAP you at least have a base level to measure any increase of

symptoms against.

### What if I am reluctant to reintroduce high FODMAP foods, is this okay?

There are both health and quality of life reasons why not reintroducing high FODMAP foods could be detrimental. Even if you feel your diet is nutritionally adequate or there is only one particular FODMAP you are reluctant to reintroduce there are other things to consider. There is some information on the reintroducing FODMAPs website to help motivate you if you are struggling to move on from the low FODMAP restriction diet. See www.reintroducingfodmaps.com and also www.rmdietetic.com for additional information.

### What if I didn't fully comply with the low FODMAP restriction phase should I still reintroduce?

If you weren't strict on avoiding high FODMAP foods when on the low FODMAP restriction diet then you may not have reduced your symptoms to a low enough level to notice any change when you start re-challenging FODMAPs. It would probably be best for you to follow the low FODMAP restriction diet for 1 or 2 more weeks and be very strict.

On the other hand if you feel you have seen a significant reduction in symptoms despite your lack of compliance then you should start the reintroduction phase as you will probably be able to notice an increase in symptoms when you re-challenge.


### *I'm quite happy eating low FODMAP vegetables and fruit so is there a need for me to reintroduce high FODMAP fruit and vegetables?*

This is a difficult one to answer without being able to assess nutritional intake. If you are eating a good variety of low FODMAP fruits and vegetables and are getting fibre from other sources such as seeds, nuts, oats and suitable cereals then your fibre and nutrient intake should be fine. However you will not be getting the potential benefits from prebiotics naturally found in certain FODMAPs such as FOS (fructo-oligosaccharides), fructans and GOS.

Also you will continue to have the problem of sticking to a restricted low FODMAP diet when you eat out making your food choices limited.

***I have been following the low FODMAP restriction diet for a long time. If I then re-challenge FODMAPs after a long period of time would this potentially make symptoms worse?***

If you have been avoiding all high FODMAP foods for longer than recommended then you may find that when you re-challenge you experience symptoms that feel worse than before you started the low FODMAP diet. It is not known why this is but it may be due to the change in gut microbiota caused by a decrease in the amount of prebiotics usually consumed when eating high FODMAP foods. This is why it is important to reintroduce FODMAPs to help prevent further gastrointestinal issues. If you have been avoiding FODMAPs for an extended period then when you re-challenge you should start with a smaller portion size than outlined in the book and then gradually increase.  Please note the severity of IBS changes over time due to the nature of the condition, therefore trying reintroduction again in the future is always a possibility.

## *Do I have to use the portion sizes recommended or can I try smaller amounts first?*

As mentioned in the question above you can start with smaller portion sizes than advised. Just make sure you follow the re-challenge protocol by gradually increasing the amount of FODMAP you are re-challenging and assessing your symptoms. You may wish to do this if you usually eat smaller portion sizes than what is outlined in the book or if you feel you need to be cautious.

## *How do I just test gluten?*

Foods that contain wheat will also contain gluten. Wheat will also contain fructans however gluten does not contain any fructans.

Trying to separate the effects of gluten from the effects of fructans is difficult. In a study that tested the effects of gluten on gut symptoms separately to fructans they used commercially available, carbohydrate-depleted wheat gluten. This study found that gluten specifically did not cause an increase in gastrointestinal symptoms. You can read the study which is open access (Accessed September 2015) http://www.gastrojournal.org/article/S0016-5085(13)00702-6/abstract

If you feel gluten is triggering symptoms then you could always re-challenge wheat and record your symptoms. You can then re-challenge non wheat foods that contain fructans such as garlic and onion. If you get symptoms only from wheat containing foods rather than vegetables containing fructans then it may be that gluten is a symptom trigger for you. This is not a definitive answer however as fructans are found in varying amounts in wheat foods, even within the same food e.g. one type or brand of bread will have higher amounts of fructans than another. The most important aspect of your health in terms of gluten is to make sure you have had a coeliac screening test to ensure you do not have coeliac disease. You must speak to your doctor or dietitian if you are unsure about this.

## *Can I try combining different high FODMAP foods in the same re-challenge?*

You should stick to the same food for the duration of the re-challenge.  So if you are testing the FODMAP GOS and have chosen chick peas then continue to use chick peas.  Do not have chick peas on day one and black beans on day two as although they are both high in GOS they will have different amounts so keeping to the same food will help control the dose of FODMAPs and allow you to better define your tolerance level.  The reintroduction phase is not an exact science so it is best to keep things simple and systematic to avoid unknown variables that may affect the outcome.

*Can I clarify that with the fructans you need to re-challenge each fructans you would want to reintroduce and cannot presume that if you are okay with bread you will also be okay with pasta? Also the large portion size of pasta is rather a lot?*

Fructans in wheat are vary variable so it makes sense to test them separately i.e. pasta is a separate re-challenge to bread. Experience shows that it is often the portion size rather than the specific FODMAP that triggers symptoms i.e. eating a larger portion of any of the FODMAPs may cause symptoms. Regarding the specific portion size, if any of the suggested portion sizes for the re-challenges seem too large or unrealistic for you they can be changed. It is the gradual increase of FODMAPs that is the important thing.

*When I start including all the tolerated FODMAPs back into my diet, how long should I stay on this*

### *before starting to reintroduce all FODMAPs into my diet?*

There is no black or white answers to this and it is best not to be to prescriptive. Additional foods should be incorporated naturally into the diet and not systematically reintroduced.  Once you know if there is a particular FODMAP that triggers symptoms you can better guess what foods may cause problems. However it is often the food combining rather than the individual FODMAPs that trigger symptoms and this will be different in everyone. Section 2 which is on Reintroducing FODMAPs helps guide you in the right direction for starting this process.  At the end of the day reintroducing FODMAPs is to help with controlling your symptoms in the long term. If you realise that a certain combination of FODMAPs triggers symptoms but you want to eat them for a special occasion then this is your decision and absolutely fine to do. The fact that you know you are likely to get symptoms from the food may actually help you control your symptoms as you know what to expect. Unlike in the past when you probably were not sure what was causing your symptoms.

## *In the tables detailing the FODMAP portion sizes what are the estimated weights for the tablespoon measures?*

To provide a guide to the estimated weights of foods you need to consume in order to gradually increase the FODMAP content a few standard rules were applied as follows:

For all beans, pulses and peas the approximate values used were;

1 tablespoon = 20g / 1oz

2 tablespoons = 50g / 2oz

4 tablespoon = 100g / 3oz

6 tablespoon = 150g / 5oz

While for nuts and seeds the approximate values used were;

1 tablespoon = 13g / ½oz

2 tablespoons = 26g / 1oz

Please note all tablespoon measures are for **heaped tablespoons** not level tablespoons.

## *Does it matter if you measure your portion sizes in grams (g) or ounces (oz.)?*

As a general rule all measures are given in grams first. These are the most accurate measures and you can use a conversion table to convert grams into the weight you need. For ease of use the book also gives weights in ounces and these are rounded up to the nearest ounce to give an estimate. For example 50g is classed as 2 ounces when to be completely accurate 60g is actually 2 ounces. These small discrepancies should not have an impact on your overall FODMAP intake and are provided to help make the reintroducing process much simpler.

# Further support

- Please email any questions you have on this book and the entire reintroduction phase of the low FODMAP diet to info@reintroducingfodmaps.com

- A complied list of frequently asked questions will be added to www.reintroducingfodmaps.com so please also check there for updates.

- If there are any changes to the FODMAP content of foods this will be updated on the website (www.reintroducingfodmaps.com) and in subsequent editions of the book.

- For further information, tips recipes, travel guides and much more on IBS and the low FODMAP diet see the blog 'Two dietitians do the low FODMAP diet' at www.rmdietetic.com

- Finally if you are finding you are unable to self-manage your IBS symptoms then please speak to your doctor or dietitian for further support.

# Acknowledgements

Written by Lee Martin RD MSc.

Data for the FODMAP content and portion sizes of foods extracted from 'The Monash University low FODMAP diet app' available to the public:

http://www.med.monash.edu/cecs/gastro/fodmap/iphone-app.html

Protocol for re-challenging FODMAPs adapted from King's College London FODMAP research teams 'Reintroducing FODMAPs' booklet, only available to registered dietitians:

www.kcl.ac.uk/fodmaps

# Contents

74520982R10044

Made in the USA
Middletown, DE
26 May 2018